MICRONEEDLING PROCEDURES FOR BEGINNERS

Comprehensive Guide To Techniques, Benefits, And Safety For Effective Skin Care And Anti-Aging Solutions

DR SAWYER DIEGO

DISCLAMER

Nothing in this book should be interpreted as medical advice; it is meant exclusively for educational reasons. Regarding their specific health issues and treatment options, readers are urged to speak with licensed healthcare professionals. The publisher and author disclaim all liability for any errors or omissions in the material provided, as well as for any negative effects that may arise from using or abusing the information. Although every attempt has been taken to guarantee that the material in this book is correct as of the date of publishing, new research may have superseded some of the content because medical knowledge is always changing. It is recommended that readers confirm the most recent medical recommendations and guidelines. The reader of this book undertakes to release the author and publisher from any claims or liabilities resulting from the use of this information, and understands and accepts the inherent risks connected with healthcare decisions.

TABLE OF CONTENTS

ABOUT THE BOOK

Understanding the tools and techniques involved in microneedling is crucial, and this book carefully navigates through various devices and methods, differentiating between DIY approaches and professional treatments. "Microneedling Procedures for Beginners" is an indispensable guide for anyone intrigued by the transformative potential of microneedling in skincare. It meticulously breaks down the intricate science and artistry behind microneedling, from its historical roots to its modern applications. It begins with a comprehensive introduction to microneedling, elucidating its numerous benefits such as skin rejuvenation, scar reduction, and overall skin health enhancement.

A notable feature of the book is its practical approach to skin preparation, which emphasizes the significance of cleansing and choosing the right skincare products to maximize treatment results. It also goes into detail about microneedling techniques, providing readers with a step-by-step guide customized for various skin concerns and body areas, making sure they understand the subtleties of choosing the right needle length, depth, and pressure application for the best results. Post-treatment care is also well-emphasized, taking readers through both short-term and long-term skincare regimens, handling side effects, and comprehending the healing process.

To ensure a safe and hygienic treatment environment, this book thoroughly discusses sterilization procedures, FDA regulations, and precautions against contamination. It also answers frequently asked questions and clarifies pain management, frequency of treatments, and suitability for different skin types, dispelling myths about do-it-yourself microneedling. Finally, it delves into advanced techniques such as combination therapies and creative applications, demonstrating the versatility of microneedling in improving aesthetic results and skin regeneration.

This book is an invaluable resource for both skincare enthusiasts and aspiring practitioners as it covers both the current state of microneedling and its future developments, making it an indispensable tool in the rapidly changing field of aesthetic dermatology. It can be used to troubleshoot common mistakes, adjust techniques, and anticipate future trends in microneedling technology.

CHAPTER ONE
MICRONEEDLING PROCEDURES OVERVIEW
MICRONEEDLING DEFINITION

Microneedling is a cosmetic procedure that involves the use of fine needles to create tiny, undetectable puncture wounds in the skin's outermost layer. These tiny wounds, known as micro-injuries, cause the skin to produce more collagen and elastin, which aids in the skin's natural healing process. By inducing this regeneration, microneedling helps to improve the texture and firmness of the skin, minimize wrinkles, scars, and stretch marks, and improve the overall appearance of the skin. The procedure can be done on different body parts, such as the face, neck, and décolletage, and is appropriate for all skin types.

Microneedling is a minimally invasive procedure that stimulates the production of collagen naturally and improves the appearance of the skin over time. A derma roller or micro needling pen is gently rolled or pressed over the skin to create controlled punctures. These micro-channels allow skincare products, like serums or creams, to penetrate deeper into the skin layers, enhancing their effectiveness. The depth of needle penetration can vary depending on the specific skin concerns being addressed, with shorter needles used for superficial treatments and longer needles for deeper scars or wrinkles.

THE ADVANTAGES OF MICRONEEDLING

In addition to improving the appearance of fine lines, wrinkles, and acne scars, microneedling can also improve the absorption and efficacy of skincare products by forming micro-channels in the skin that allow active ingredients to penetrate deeply.

These are just a few of the many benefits that microneedling offers for skin rejuvenation and enhancement. One of the main benefits is that it can stimulate the production of collagen and elastin, which helps to tighten and firm the skin.

Another important advantage of microneedling is that it can be used to treat a wide range of skin issues, such as hyperpigmentation, enlarged pores, and stretch marks. Microneedling also helps to even out skin tone and texture by stimulating cell turnover and enhancing skin regeneration. Finally, because the procedure is quick and doesn't require much downtime in comparison to more invasive treatments, it is appropriate for people with hectic schedules.

COMPREHENDING THE TOOLS AND TECHNIQUES OF MICRONEEDLING

Microneedling pens and dermarollers are two common types of microneedling tools that are used to create precise micro-channels in the skin. Microneedling pens have an oscillating motorized tip, while derma rollers are cylindrical drum studded with tiny needles that are rolled across the skin's surface. Both types of tools come in different needle lengths, ranging from 0.5 to 3 millimeters, allowing for customization based on the particular skin concerns and treatment area.

Home microneedling kits are also available for personal use, although they typically feature shorter needles and require careful adherence to hygiene and technique for optimal results. Professional microneedling sessions are often performed in dermatology or cosmetic clinics by trained practitioners to ensure safety and efficacy. Microneedling techniques involve gently rolling or pressing the device over the skin in different directions, ensuring even coverage and controlled penetration depth.

SAFETY FACTORS TO CONSIDER WITH MICRONEEDLING

Even though microneedling is generally thought to be safe when carried out by qualified professionals or with approved home devices, there are a few things to keep in mind to reduce the risks: using high-quality serums or skincare products that are recommended for microneedling is vital to prevent adverse reactions or allergies; sterilizing microneedling tools properly is crucial to prevent infections because the procedure creates micro-injuries that could introduce bacteria into the skin.

Sun protection is essential after microneedling treatments, as the skin may be more sensitive to UV radiation. Speaking with a dermatologist or skincare professional before undergoing microneedling can help assess skin suitability and address any concerns regarding the procedure's safety and effectiveness for particular skin types or conditions. People with active skin infections, such as acne or eczema, should avoid microneedling until these conditions have resolved to prevent exacerbation.

HOW YOU CAN BENEFIT FROM THIS BOOK

In addition to covering important topics like understanding microneedling tools, choosing appropriate needle lengths based on skin concerns, and outlining step-by-step techniques for effective treatment, this book serves as a comprehensive guide for beginners to micro needling, offering practical insights into the procedure's benefits, techniques, and safety considerations. It also discusses how microneedling stimulates collagen production, which improves skin texture and reduces signs of aging.

Additionally, this resource highlights the significance of appropriate skin care and post-treatment care regimens to optimize microneedling outcomes and preserve skin health. It also offers helpful advice on selecting appropriate serums or creams to optimize treatment efficacy and clarifies common questions or misconceptions regarding microneedling. Whether you're thinking about professional treatments or investigating at-home options, this book gives you the information and assurance you need to start your microneedling journey efficiently and securely.

CHAPTER TWO

FUNDAMENTALS OF MICRONEEDLING

THE MEANING AND BACKGROUND OF MICRONEEDLING

Collagen induction therapy, or microneedling, is a minimally invasive cosmetic procedure that uses fine needles to create tiny punctures in the skin. These micro-injuries encourage the skin's natural healing processes, resulting in increased production of collagen and elastin.

The main goals of this treatment are to improve the appearance of scars, texture, and overall appearance of the skin. The idea behind microneedling dates back to ancient times when different types of skin puncturing were used for rejuvenation, albeit in more primitive forms.

Microneedling's modern history started in the mid-1990s when it was developed as a controlled way to induce collagen remodeling without severely damaging the epidermis. Originally used to treat wrinkles and scars, microneedling has expanded to address a variety of dermatological issues, such as hyperpigmentation and stretch marks. Today, it is considered a highly adaptable treatment that can be used for a variety of skin types and conditions.

Microneedling is a versatile procedure that can be customized based on the depth of needle penetration and the specific skin concerns being addressed. It works on the principle of controlled injury to the skin, triggering the release of growth factors and stimulating the production of collagen and elastin. Over time, this process helps to repair and rejuvenate the skin from within, leading to improved texture, firmness, and elasticity.

THE SCIENCE OF MICRONEEDLING

Microneedling's science is based on the skin's natural healing response: tiny punctures create micro-channels that temporarily disrupt the barrier function; this controlled injury sets off a cascade of events that lead to wound healing, beginning with the release of growth factors and cytokines, which are signaling molecules that draw immune cells to the site of injury and encourage tissue regeneration.

One of the main effects of microneedling is the induction of collagen, the main structural protein in the skin that gives strength and support.

New collagen fibers are synthesized to replace old, damaged collagen as the skin repairs the micro-injuries caused by microneedling, which not only improves skin firmness and elasticity but also helps to smooth out fine lines, wrinkles, and scars over time.

While superficial treatments concentrate on improving product absorption and superficial skin rejuvenation, deeper penetration targets dermal layers where collagen production is stimulated more significantly. The science behind microneedling underscores its effectiveness in treating a variety of skin concerns, from acne scars to signs of aging, by utilizing the skin's natural ability to heal and regenerate.

MICRONEEDLING DEVICE TYPES

Pen devices use a reciprocating motion to deliver precise, vertical needle penetration into the skin; roller devices use a cylindrical drum studded with needles, which are rolled over the skin's surface to create micro-channels.

Microneedling devices come in a variety of forms, from basic roller devices with multiple needles to sophisticated motorized pens equipped with adjustable needle depths and precision controls.

In addition, advanced pen devices may incorporate technologies like radiofrequency or LED light therapy to further enhance collagen induction and skin rejuvenation. Motorized microneedling pens offer advantages like adjustable needle depth settings, allowing practitioners to tailor treatments based on individual skin needs and conditions.

These pens often come with disposable needle cartridges to ensure sterility and minimize the risk of cross-contamination.

Understanding the differences between these devices helps individuals and practitioners choose the most appropriate option for achieving desired aesthetic outcomes. Each type of microneedling device has its unique benefits and considerations.

For example, roller devices are usually less expensive and easier to use at home, but they may be less precise than motorized pens used in professional settings. Professional-grade pens offer greater control over treatment parameters, making them suitable for addressing specific skin concerns under the guidance of trained skincare professionals.

WHAT SEPARATES PROFESSIONAL AND DO-IT-YOURSELF MICRONEEDLING

The main differences between professional microneedling and DIY (do-it-yourself) treatments are safety, efficacy, and precision. DIY microneedling usually entails using derma rollers or handheld rollers at home under professional supervision; although these devices can enhance the absorption of skincare products and the texture of the skin on the surface, they lack the sterility and precision of professional-grade equipment used in clinical settings.

Professional treatments also adhere to strict hygiene protocols and may incorporate additional technologies like radiofrequency or growth factor serums to enhance treatment outcomes.

Trained skincare professionals, such as dermatologists or licensed aestheticians, perform professional microneedling treatments using advanced motorized pens with adjustable needle depths.

These devices ensure controlled needle penetration at optimal depths tailored to individual skin concerns, minimizing the risk of complications like infection or uneven results.

Another important consideration that sets professional microneedling apart from DIY is efficacy. Although DIY devices can produce noticeable results over time, professional treatments frequently yield more significant and consistent results because of the precise needle penetration and complementary skincare protocols. Professionals can also offer customized recommendations based on the patient's skin type, medical history, and treatment goals, ensuring safe and effective results with minimal downtime.

Knowing the distinctions between professional and do-it-yourself microneedling allows people to make well-informed decisions about their aesthetic procedures and skincare regimens. Professional procedures provide better safety, accuracy, and effectiveness for treating a variety of skin issues under the guidance of a professional. DIY options are more convenient and accessible.

COMMON MISCONCEPTIONS AND MYTHS REGARDING MICRONEEDLING

Even though topical numbing creams are usually applied before the procedure to minimize discomfort, there are many myths surrounding microneedling, which has become more and more popular in recent years.

One such myth is that the procedure is painful. In reality, most people find the sensation during microneedling to be mild, tingling or prickling.

Another myth is that microneedling is only good for wrinkles. Although it stimulates collagen production, which improves fine lines and wrinkles, it also targets other skin concerns like acne scars, hyperpigmentation, and uneven skin texture. Because of its versatility, microneedling can be used to treat a variety of dermatological issues outside of signs of aging.

Another myth is that microneedling requires a lot of downtime.

In reality, most people only experience very little downtime following the procedure. The skin may feel sensitive or appear slightly red after the procedure, but these effects usually go away in a day or two, allowing people to resume their regular activities after the procedure as long as they use proper skincare.

It's also a common misconception that darker skin tones cannot benefit from microneedling. Although skin type and pigmentation levels affect treatment parameters, microneedling is safe for all skin types when proper adjustments are made to needle depth and post-care protocols.

Speaking with a qualified skincare professional guarantees customized treatment plans that prioritize safety and efficacy for a range of skin tones.

By debunking these myths, people can make well-informed decisions about microneedling treatments that are grounded in realistic expectations and accurate information.

People can confidently explore microneedling as a viable option for achieving smoother, rejuvenated skin by understanding the science behind the procedure and its broad range of applications.

CHAPTER THREE

PREPARING THE SKIN FOR MICRONEEDLING

THE VALUE OF SKIN PREPARATION

Ensuring the safety and efficacy of microneedling requires proper skin preparation. Exfoliating your skin gently can promote cell turnover, which can improve the overall texture and appearance of your skin after treatment.

It can also help remove impurities, excess oil, and makeup residues that can interfere with the microneedling process. Finally, proper skin preparation helps enhance the penetration of the microneedles into the skin, allowing for better absorption of serums and promoting optimal results.

Furthermore, clean, well-prepped skin lowers the chance of introducing bacteria or other contaminants into the microchannels created by the needles, which makes it easier to minimize the risk of infection and irritation during microneedling. This preparation step is crucial for individuals who want to achieve smoother, more radiant skin and maximize the benefits of microneedling treatments.

To guarantee that your skin is resilient and plump before the procedure, it is also important to properly hydrate it. This will not only help you feel less uncomfortable during the procedure but will also speed up your recovery afterward.

In summary, taking the time to properly prepare your skin in advance will guarantee that your microneedling session is successful and that you get the most out of your treatment.

HYGIENE AND CLEANING PROCEDURES

It is essential to thoroughly cleanse your skin before microneedling. Use lukewarm water and pat dry with a clean towel to prevent irritation or damage. Wash your face with a gentle cleanser to remove dirt, oil, and any leftover makeup.

This step ensures that the microneedles can penetrate the skin effectively without encountering barriers like excess oil or debris.

Ensuring that your hands, the microneedling device, and any other tools used are completely sanitized is crucial to preventing infections and complications during microneedling. This lowers the possibility of introducing bacteria into the microchannels created by the needles, which could result in infections or other unfavorable reactions.

Following these cleansing and hygiene practices not only prepares your skin for microneedling but also helps maintain its health and integrity throughout the procedure. Avoid using harsh exfoliants or products that may irritate the skin after cleansing, as this can increase sensitivity during microneedling. Instead, opt for gentle skincare products that are suitable for your skin type.

SELECTING THE APPROPRIATE SKINCARE PRODUCTS

To get the best results from microneedling, choose the right products for skin preparation. Avoid products with harsh chemicals or exfoliants that could irritate the skin and impair its barrier function. Instead, look for gentle cleansers that effectively remove impurities without stripping the skin of its natural oils.

Apart from using cleansers, think about using lightweight, non-comedogenic hydrating serums or moisturizers to help restore moisture and prepare the skin for microneedling.

This will help improve the absorption of active ingredients during the procedure, and certain ingredients, like hyaluronic acid, can be especially helpful for plumping the skin and minimizing the appearance of fine lines and wrinkles.

Selecting the right products guarantees that your skin is in optimal condition to undergo the microneedling procedure safely and effectively. If you have specific skin concerns, such as acne or hyperpigmentation, speak with a skincare professional to find the best products for your needs. They can recommend targeted treatments or serums that address your specific skin concerns while effectively preparing your skin for microneedling.

SKIN TYPES THAT CAN BE MICRONEEDLES

A versatile treatment option for many, microneedling is generally suitable for a wide range of skin conditions and concerns.

It can effectively improve the appearance of wrinkles, fine lines, acne scars, enlarged pores, and uneven skin texture. By creating micro-injuries, the procedure stimulates the production of collagen, which helps to rejuvenate the skin over time and promote a smoother, more youthful complexion.

Microneedling works best for people with generally healthy skin and reasonable expectations.

To make sure the treatment is safe and effective, it's important to speak with a qualified skincare professional to evaluate your skin type, sensitivity, and any underlying conditions before deciding if microneedling is right for you.

Microneedling is a great treatment for many skin conditions, but it may not be the best option for people with rosacea, eczema, active acne, or other inflammatory skin conditions, as these conditions can make the procedure more prone to complications or irritation.

It's important to talk to a professional about your skincare objectives and medical history to find out if microneedling is the best option for your particular skin concerns.

WARNING SIGNS AND EXCLUSIONS

To guarantee a safe and successful treatment outcome, it is important to be informed about any possible precautions and contraindications before undergoing microneedling. Patients who have a history of keloid scars or hypertrophic scars might not be good candidates for microneedling because it could make these conditions worse.

Likewise, pregnant patients or those with active infections or skin conditions in the treatment area should postpone microneedling until these conditions have resolved.

Your skincare professional will evaluate your medical history and skin condition to determine whether microneedling is appropriate and safe for you. Post-care instructions, such as avoiding sun exposure and applying soothing skincare products, help minimize the risk of adverse reactions and support optimal healing after microneedling. It is important to disclose any medications you are taking, especially blood thinners or topical treatments, as these may affect the suitability of microneedling for your skin.

Prioritizing safety and suitability allows you to get the desired results from microneedling while minimizing potential risks and complications. By being aware of these precautions and contraindications, you can make educated decisions about microneedling and ensure that you undergo the treatment under the supervision of a qualified skincare professional.

CHAPTER FOUR

TECHNIQUES FOR MICRONEEDLING

A COMPREHENSIVE GUIDE TO MICRONEEDLING PROCEDURES

To perform microneedling effectively, the skin must first be thoroughly cleaned and, if desired, numbing cream applied to minimize discomfort. Next, depending on the skin concern being addressed, choose an appropriate needle length (usually ranging from 0.5 to 2.5 millimeters): longer needles are suitable for treating scars and deep wrinkles, while shorter needles are used for general skin rejuvenation. Microneedling is a minimally invasive cosmetic procedure that involves puncturing the skin with fine needles to stimulate collagen production and improve skin texture.

Maintaining constant pressure to ensure even penetration without causing excessive trauma, hold the microneedling device at a 90-degree angle to the skin and roll or stamp gently in horizontal, vertical, and diagonal directions across the treatment area. After the procedure, apply a soothing serum or moisturizer to aid in recovery and promote healing. Avoid vigorous exercise and the sun for at least 24 hours post-treatment to prevent irritation and promote optimal results. Microneedling can help achieve smoother, firmer skin with improved tone and texture with regular sessions spaced several weeks apart.

CHOOSING THE RIGHT NEEDLE LENGTH FOR YOUR SKIN CONCERNS

For fine lines, shallow acne scars, and general skin rejuvenation, needles between 0.5 and 1.0 millimeters are recommended. These shorter needles promote collagen production and improve the absorption of topical skincare products, leading to smoother and more radiant skin over time. Selecting the appropriate needle length for microneedling is essential for effectively and safely addressing specific skin concerns.

Longer needles, 1.5 to 2.5 millimeters, are needed for deeper skin issues like deep wrinkles, stretch marks, and prominent scars. These lengths go deeper into the dermis, stimulating cellular turnover and a more significant collagen response, but it's important to use longer needles cautiously to avoid excessive pain or skin damage. If you're new to microneedling, always start with shorter needles and gradually increase the length as you become more comfortable with the procedure and understand your skin's response.

STRATEGIES FOR VARIOUS FACE AND BODY AREAS

For the face, divide the treatment area into sections and work methodically from the forehead down to the chin. Use gentle, overlapping motions to cover each section evenly, adjusting the angle and pressure of the device as needed for sensitive areas like around the eyes or lips. Different microneedling techniques are used depending on the area of the body or face being treated to ensure optimal results and safety.

For more delicate areas like the neck or décolletage, use shorter needles and lighter pressure to reduce the risk of irritation or injury. Always use a soothing serum or moisturizer to calm the skin and support the healing process after treatment. Focus on one area at a time and use longer strokes to ensure comprehensive coverage. Maintain a steady hand and consistent pressure to avoid uneven results or discomfort.

KNOWING PRESSURE AND DEPTH

Since depth describes how deeply the needles penetrate the skin's layers and pressure describes the force used during the procedure, these two factors have a significant impact on the effectiveness and safety of microneedling.

You should adjust the depth settings on your micro needling device based on the skin concern and area being treated, using shallower depths for superficial issues and deeper depths for more profound skin imperfections.

To achieve optimal microneedling results safely, always prioritize safety and follow manufacturer guidelines regarding depth settings and pressure levels. Starting with low to moderate pressure and gradually increasing as you become more experienced and comfortable with the process will help ensure even needle penetration without causing unnecessary trauma to the skin. Too much pressure can result in discomfort or bruising, while too little pressure may result in ineffective treatment.

ADVICE FOR GETTING THE BEST OUTCOMES

The best outcomes from microneedling depend on how well the skin is prepared and how well the post-treatment care is followed. To minimize discomfort, use a numbing cream if you have a low pain threshold.

Before beginning, thoroughly clean the skin to remove any makeup, dirt, or oil, as these can interfere with needle penetration and efficacy.

To prevent uneven results or overstimulation of specific areas, make sure you maintain a steady hand and consistent motion throughout the microneedling area. After the procedure, hydrate the skin and support its recovery by applying a calming serum or moisturizer enriched with soothing ingredients such as hyaluronic acid or aloe vera. Refrain from sun exposure and strenuous activities for at least 24 hours following the procedure to prevent irritation and encourage optimal healing.

You can reap the benefits of microneedling for smoother, healthier-looking skin by following these tips and sticking to a strict skincare routine. Microneedling works best when you schedule regular sessions spaced several weeks apart. You'll notice improvements in skin texture, tone, and firmness over time as well as cumulative benefits. You'll also need to monitor your skin's response to each session and make necessary adjustments to your technique or needle length.

CHAPTER FIVE

RECUPERATION AND AFTERCARE

QUICK POST-TREATMENT MONITORING

Immediately following microneedling, proper healing and outcomes depend on proper post-treatment care. To start, the treated area should be gently cleansed to get rid of any leftover numbing cream, blood, or lymphatic fluid. Mild cleanser and tepid water should be used; avoid using harsh products that could irritate the skin. Finally, the skin should be patted dry with a clean towel, being careful not to rub or apply pressure.

After cleansing, use a calming serum or moisturizer that your skincare specialist has recommended. This will help to hydrate the skin and improve the skin's ability to absorb active ingredients after treatment. Avoid using thick creams or products with potent active ingredients as they can irritate the skin. If the treatment was done during the day, you should apply sunscreen to protect the skin from UV rays.

Follow these guidelines to support the skin's healing process and minimize the risk of complications during the first 24-48 hours following microneedling. Avoid activities that could raise skin temperature or cause excessive sweating, such as intense exercise or hot showers. You should also avoid direct sun exposure, swimming in chlorinated pools, and using saunas or steam rooms during this initial healing period.

EXTENDED SKIN CARE PROTOCOLS

After microneedling, you should create a long-term skincare routine to preserve and improve the results. Use mild cleansers and hydrating serums every day to keep the skin clear and hydrated. Hyaluronic acid and peptide-based products can help with skin regeneration by encouraging the production of collagen and hydration.

Sunscreen with a broad spectrum SPF of 30 or higher should be used daily to prevent pigmentation problems and premature aging, both of which can be made worse by sun exposure. Use sunscreen liberally every morning, even on overcast days, and reapply as needed throughout the day to preserve the benefits of microneedling.

Add retinol or vitamin C serums to your nighttime routine to increase the production of collagen and improve the texture of your skin. These ingredients also help to minimize fine lines, improve overall skin clarity, and fade hyperpigmentation. Since consistency is important when it comes to skincare, follow your regimen religiously to get the most out of microneedling in the long run and maintain healthy, glowing skin.

HANDLING RISKS AND SIDE EFFECTS

A good microneedling experience requires an understanding of the risks and possible side effects. Mild redness and swelling are common right after the procedure and go away in a few hours to a day. You can minimize swelling and discomfort by applying an ice pack or cold compress wrapped in a clean cloth.

Since picking at scabs or peeling skin can exacerbate the condition and increase the risk of infection or scarring, try to resist the urge to scratch and instead apply a light moisturizer to relieve the irritation. Temporary flaking or dryness of the skin is normal during the healing process, so it's crucial to stay properly hydrated with non-comedogenic products.

Keep an eye out for symptoms of infection, such as increased redness, warmth, or pus-like discharge from the treated area. If you notice any of these, get in touch with your skincare specialist right away for additional assessment and care. You can reduce risks and get the best results from microneedling if you follow post-care instructions and stay aware of potential complications.

UNDERSTANDING THE TYPICAL HEALING PROCESS

It is helpful to know what to expect from the normal healing process following microneedling to ensure proper aftercare.

Following treatment, the skin may appear red or flushed, resembling mild sunburn; this usually goes away in 24-48 hours. Some people may experience minor pinpoint bleeding or bruising at the treatment sites, but these side effects are normal and go away quickly.

The skin will feel tighter and slightly rougher to the touch during the next few days as it starts to regenerate. This is an indication that collagen production is starting, which will eventually result in smoother, firmer skin. As the skin heals, you might notice gradual improvements in texture, tone, and overall radiance, with full results showing up in a few weeks to months.

Consistency in skincare and adherence to post-care instructions play key roles in achieving the desired outcomes from microneedling. If you have concerns about your skin's appearance or your healing progress, speak with your skin care professional for guidance and assurance.

It's important to be patient during the healing process and avoid expecting immediate dramatic changes.

WHEN TO SET UP ADDITIONAL MEETINGS

Your skincare professional will evaluate your skin's response to the initial treatment and recommend an appropriate schedule for follow-up sessions. The best time for follow-up sessions after microneedling depends on the specific condition being addressed and the goals of each treatment; generally, 4-6 weeks apart is recommended to achieve cumulative benefits and maximize results.

Regular communication with your skincare provider ensures that treatment plans are customized to your skin's unique needs and desired outcomes. Follow-up sessions help maintain and build upon the improvements achieved with microneedling, stimulating ongoing collagen production and skin rejuvenation. If you are targeting specific concerns like acne scars or fine lines, additional sessions may be necessary to achieve optimal results.

You can maintain long-term improvements in skin tone, texture, and appearance by keeping follow-up appointments at the prescribed intervals. Ask questions or voice any concerns you may have about the procedure or the results at your appointments to make sure you are getting the most out of microneedling.

CHAPTER SIX

ADVANTAGES AND OUTCOMES OF MICRO-NEEDLING

BENEFITS FOR SKIN: PIGMENTATION, ACNE SCARS, AND ANTI-AGING

Numerous skin benefits are associated with microneedling, which makes it a flexible treatment for a variety of concerns, including anti-aging, pigmentation issues, and acne scars.

One of the main advantages of microneedling is that it is an effective way to stimulate the production of collagen, which is necessary for skin elasticity and firmness but diminishes with age, resulting in wrinkles and fine lines.

Microneedling works by inducing tiny punctures in the skin, which stimulates the body's natural healing process and produces collagen and elastin, resulting in smoother, firmer skin over time, minimizing the appearance of wrinkles and fine lines.

For acne scars, microneedling works wonders as well. It breaks down old scar tissue and encourages the creation of new collagen and elastin, which results in smoother skin texture and less scarring after several sessions. In terms of pigmentation problems, such as sun spots or melasma, microneedling improves topical treatment absorption and promotes even distribution of melanin, which eventually leads to a more balanced complexion with less pigmentation.

This minimally invasive procedure uses a device with tiny needles to create controlled micro-injuries, so there is minimal discomfort and downtime. Overall, microneedling is a good treatment for a variety of skin concerns, with noticeable improvements in skin texture, tone, and overall youthfulness with regular sessions. Most skin types and tones can benefit from microneedling, though consulting with a dermatologist or skincare professional is advised to determine the best approach for individual skin concerns.

ANTICIPATED OUTCOMES WITH TIME

Anyone thinking about getting microneedling should know what to expect from the procedure over time. Patients can experience slight improvements in skin tone and texture following the first session because of increased collagen production and better skincare product absorption. However, noticeable improvements usually occur after a series of sessions spaced a few weeks apart.

Throughout treatments—which typically last three to six sessions, depending on the severity of skin issues—people can anticipate gradual improvements in skin texture, a decrease in acne scars, and an evening out of pigmentation. As collagen continues to rebuild, fine lines and wrinkles gradually disappear, leaving behind smoother, firmer skin that looks younger.

While deep scars or extensive pigmentation may require additional treatments or complementary procedures, it's important to manage realistic expectations. Microneedling can produce dramatic improvements, especially in skin texture and tone. Over time, optimal results depend on consistent treatment sessions and adherence to post-procedure care instructions.

REASONABLE ANTICIPATIONS FOR MICRONEEDLING

Setting reasonable expectations for microneedling is essential to achieving a satisfactory result. Although the procedure can significantly improve pigmentation, acne scars, and skin texture, individual skin conditions and adherence to recommended treatment plans can affect the outcome.

Throughout several sessions, microneedling can effectively reduce the appearance of fine lines and wrinkles, improve skin texture, and diminish scars and pigmentation. However, it may be necessary to undergo additional treatments or combination therapies tailored to specific skin concerns to eliminate deep scars or extensive pigmentation.

Results become more evident as collagen continues to repair over several weeks following each treatment, with skin appearing smoother, firmer, and more luminous. Patients may anticipate some redness and minor swelling immediately following each session, which usually resolves within a few days.

Understanding the potential benefits and limitations of microneedling allows patients to approach the treatment with confidence, knowing what to expect throughout the process. Consulting with a qualified dermatologist or skincare professional is essential to assess skin suitability for microneedling and to establish realistic expectations based on individual skin concerns and goals.

USING MICRONEEDLING IN CONJUNCTION WITH OTHER THERAPIES

Since microneedling creates microchannels in the skin, combining it with other skincare treatments can improve overall results and address multiple skin concerns at once.

Topical skincare products applied during or right after the procedure will absorb and work much better because of this.

To further enhance skin elasticity and stimulate collagen production for anti-aging purposes, microneedling can be combined with serums containing hyaluronic acid, peptides, or growth factors. This combination amplifies the rejuvenating effects of microneedling, promoting smoother, plumper skin with reduced fine lines and wrinkles.

Combining microneedling with laser therapies or chemical peels can produce more comprehensive results when targeting specific skin issues such as acne scars or hyperpigmentation. Laser therapies, like fractional laser resurfacing, can further enhance collagen production and skin texture, while chemical peels help to exfoliate the skin and improve overall complexion.

To create a customized treatment plan based on each patient's unique concerns and objectives, it is imperative to speak with a skincare specialist. Patients can achieve more profound and durable improvements in their skin's texture, tone, and overall youthfulness by combining microneedling with complementary treatments.

REFERENCES AND ACHIEVEMENTS

Examining patient testimonials and success stories from people who have had microneedling can give important information about the efficacy and outcomes of the procedure. After a series of microneedling sessions, many patients report notable improvements in skin texture, a decrease in acne scars, and an improvement in pigmentation issues.

Success stories highlight the treatment's ability to rejuvenate and revitalize the skin, resulting in a more youthful and radiant complexion over time. Testimonials frequently highlight the gradual yet noticeable changes in skin appearance, with smoother texture, diminished fine lines, and increased firmness being common benefits.

Feedback highlighting the minimal discomfort during the procedure and the relatively short downtime that makes microneedling a convenient option for busy lifestyles is often provided by others who have had the procedure done. Real-life experiences shared by others who have had the procedure done can help prospective patients understand what to expect during and after the treatment process.

Those who are thinking about getting microneedling can become more confident in the procedure's effectiveness and possible advantages for their skin issues by reading through testimonials and success stories. Speaking with a skincare expert and talking about personal objectives can help to further define expectations and guarantee a customized strategy for reaching desired skincare outcomes.

CHAPTER SEVEN

HYGIENE AND SAFETY PROCEDURES

STERILIZATION AND A CLEAN ENVIRONMENT ARE IMPORTANT

Before beginning any microneedling session, it is imperative to thoroughly sterilize all tools. This includes micro needling devices, derma rollers, and any other equipment that will come into contact with the skin. Sterilization can be achieved through methods such as autoclaving, chemical disinfection, or using sterile disposable tools. Sterilization prevents the introduction of harmful bacteria or pathogens that could lead to infections or other complications during the procedure.

Keeping the workspace clear of dust, debris, and other contaminants that could compromise the procedure's sterility also helps reduce the risk of cross-contamination. Disposable barriers, such as sterile drapes or covers for surfaces, can further enhance cleanliness.

Additionally, proper hand hygiene is essential for anyone performing or assisting in microneedling procedures. Hands should be thoroughly washed with soap and water, or sanitized with alcohol-based hand rubs, before and after each treatment session.

In addition to ensuring patient safety, a sterile and clean environment can improve the efficacy of microneedling treatments. Practitioners can give their clients a safer and more dependable procedure, promoting better outcomes and lowering the risk of complications, by strictly adhering to sterilization protocols and maintaining cleanliness throughout the procedure.

FDA GUIDELINES AND DEVICES FOR MICRONEEDLING

The FDA classifies microneedling devices based on their intended use and the level of risk associated with their use; devices marketed for personal or home use may fall under different classifications than those intended for professional use in medical settings.

It is important to use FDA-cleared or FDA-approved devices, as these have undergone rigorous testing to ensure their safety and effectiveness. Practitioners and enthusiasts alike should be aware of the regulations about microneedling devices from the FDA.

The FDA forbids making false or deceptive claims about the advantages or outcomes of using microneedling devices, which protects consumers from dishonest marketing practices and guarantees that they are informed about the procedure's possible risks and benefits. Practitioners should also be aware of these regulations regarding advertising and claims made about microneedling devices.

Staying up to date on regulatory updates and changes is crucial for maintaining compliance and upholding professional standards in microneedling practice. Practitioners can provide their clients confidence in the safety and efficacy of the treatment by following FDA regulations, which guarantee that they are using safe and effective microneedling devices.

PREVENTING INFECTIONS AND CONTAMINATION

Reusable devices should be properly sterilized between uses by established protocols. Contamination and infections are major concerns in microneedling procedures, making infection control practices paramount. To minimize the risk of contamination, practitioners should use sterile disposable needles or cartridges for each treatment session.

To minimize the risk of infection, it is also crucial to properly prepare the skin. To help create a clean canvas for the procedure and lower the chance of introducing contaminants into the skin during needling, the skin should be thoroughly cleansed with an antiseptic solution before microneedling.

Keep a sterile field throughout the treatment session to reduce the risk of infections and ensure patient safety. During the procedure, practitioners should wear sterile gloves and avoid touching non-sterile surfaces or objects that could potentially transfer bacteria to the skin.

A safe and successful microneedling treatment requires practitioners to be vigilant in maintaining cleanliness and following proper sterilization protocols. By strictly adhering to infection control practices, practitioners can reduce the risk of complications and promote optimal outcomes for their clients.

SAFE MANAGEMENT AND DISCARDMENT OF MICRONEEDLING EQUIPMENT

After each use, disposable needles or cartridges should be carefully disposed of in designated sharps containers to help prevent accidental needle sticks and ensure that used needles are safely contained. Proper handling and disposal of microneedling tools are essential to maintaining safety and preventing contamination.

Before being used again, reusable microneedling devices should be thoroughly cleaned with detergent and water and then sterilized using techniques like autoclaving or chemical disinfection, as directed by the manufacturer. This ensures that the devices are free of dangerous pathogens and prepared for safe reuse.

To maintain a sterile environment and lower the risk of cross-contamination between clients, practitioners should also make sure that all additional equipment used during micro needling, such as derma rollers or skin preparation instruments, is cleaned and sanitized between usage.

Practitioners can maintain high standards of safety and hygiene in their practices by enforcing strict protocols for handling and disposing of microneedling tools. Among the most important measures to prevent infections and enhance the general safety and well-being of clients receiving microneedling treatments are the appropriate disposal of sharps and the thorough sterilization of reusable devices.

SPEAKING WITH A QUALIFIED DERMATOLOGIST

A professional dermatologist can analyze skin issues, discuss treatment goals, and offer appropriate micro needling procedures or alternatives based on individual needs, therefore speaking with one before undergoing micro needling is strongly recommended to guarantee suitability and safety.

To determine any contraindications or factors that may affect the safety or effectiveness of microneedling, the dermatologist will review the patient's medical history during the consultation. These conditions may include eczema, psoriasis, active breakouts of acne, or recent skin infections, which may call for special consideration or alternative treatments.

To maximize outcomes and minimize potential side effects, dermatologists can also offer customized guidance on pre- and post-care routines. This can include suggestions for skincare products, sun protection, and follow-up appointments to track progress and make necessary adjustments to treatment plans.

Professional dermatologists provide knowledge about skin health and treatment options, so people can make well-informed decisions about microneedling and ensure that the procedure is safe and effective for their particular skin concerns. Their advice can also improve the overall experience and results of microneedling treatments.

CHAPTER EIGHT

FREQUENTLY ASKED QUESTIONS

CONTROLLING PAIN DURING MICRONEEDLING

Despite its efficacy in skin rejuvenation, microneedling can be uncomfortable, particularly for novices. Topical numbing creams with lidocaine or prilocaine are frequently prescribed to control pain during microneedling procedures. These creams are applied to the treatment area before the session to minimize the sensation of needle pricks.

It is important to adhere to the manufacturer's instructions regarding application timing and quantity to achieve effective numbing without negative side effects.

Using cooling devices or ice packs helps numb the skin's surface and minimize discomfort during the microneedling procedure. Cooling the skin both before and after the procedure can also minimize redness and swelling, improving overall comfort level after treatment.

Additionally, microneedling practitioners frequently modify the depth of the needles based on the targeted area and the patient's pain threshold; deeper penetration of the needles can produce more noticeable results but may be more uncomfortable initially.

It is important to discuss your concerns and pain threshold with your skincare professional to customize the procedure to your comfort level and achieve the best possible results for your skin.

REGULARITY OF MICRONEEDLING TREATMENTS

The number of microneedling sessions varies based on the specific skin concerns and treatment objectives. However, experts generally advise 4 to 6 weeks between treatments to give the skin time to heal and regenerate. This allows the collagen production that is stimulated by microneedling to take effect and gradually improve skin tone and texture.

A course of 4 to 6 sessions may be suggested initially for those targeting specific skin issues, such as fine lines or acne scars. Maintenance treatments every 3 to 6 months can help sustain the improvements after the desired results are achieved, but the precise frequency should be determined in consultation with a dermatologist or licensed skincare professional based on your skin's response and ongoing skincare regimen.

Following the suggested treatment plan is crucial to prevent overstimulating the skin or interfering with its natural healing process.

Regular, spaced-out sessions facilitate progressive, long-lasting improvements in skin texture and appearance without placing undue strain on the skin barrier.

IMPACTS ON VARIOUS SKIN TYPES (DRY, OILY, AND SENSITIVE)

Sensitive, oily, and dry skin types can all react differently to microneedling. After treatment, sensitive skin types may experience increased redness and mild irritation, but these side effects usually go away in a few days. Using gentle skincare products and avoiding harsh ingredients can help minimize sensitivity after microneedling.

Microneedling may help reduce excess oil production and refine pore size over time for oily skin types. Post-treatment care is important to prevent breakouts and clogged pores, so use non-comedogenic moisturizers and avoid heavy oils.

After microneedling, dry skin types may feel temporarily flaky or dry after the procedure, especially if they are not moisturized enough. Hydrating serums and moisturizers rich in emollients can help maintain moisture levels and restore the function of the skin barrier, resulting in faster healing and better outcomes.

Knowing how various skin types react to microneedling enables skincare professionals to effectively customize treatment plans; matching skincare products and aftercare advice to individual skin needs guarantees a happy clientele and amplifies the long-term advantages of microneedling procedures.

DANGERS OF DO-IT-YOURSELF MICRONEEDLING AT HOME

Professional microneedling devices are designed with safety features and sterile needles to minimize these risks, ensuring controlled and effective treatment outcomes.

DIY microneedling at home carries significant risks and is generally discouraged by skincare professionals. Using non-sterile needles or inadequate techniques can lead to infections, scarring, and skin damage.

DIY microneedling carries a risk of infection as well as the possibility of uneven or excessive needle penetration, which can cause skin trauma instead of the desired stimulation of collagen. Professionals are trained to perform microneedling safely and effectively, knowing the right depth and technique for various skin concerns.

In addition, incorrect post-care after DIY microneedling can worsen side effects including redness, swelling, and sensitivity to the sun. Skincare professionals monitor skin reactions and offer customized aftercare instructions to maximize healing and reduce issues after treatment.

A licensed dermatologist or skincare professional trained in microneedling techniques is the best person to consult for safe and effective microneedling treatments. They can evaluate your skin condition, suggest appropriate treatment plans, and make sure the procedure is carried out correctly to produce the desired results of skin rejuvenation.

TAKING CARE OF THE PAIN AND NEEDLES FEAR

Pre-treatment consultation allows for discussion of fears and exploration of pain management options tailored to individual needs. Understanding and addressing fear of pain and needles is crucial for ensuring a comfortable microneedling experience. Skincare professionals can offer various strategies to minimize anxiety and discomfort during the procedure.

During microneedling, distraction techniques like deep breathing exercises, music, or positive imagery can help deflect attention from the sensations of the needles. Aromatherapy or the creation of a calm environment in the treatment room can further encourage relaxation and lower anxiety levels.

Additionally, selecting a certified and experienced skincare specialist for microneedling procedures fosters trust in the safety and effectiveness of the procedure.

Practitioners adept at comfort enhancement and patient communication can greatly reduce anxiety and guarantee a satisfying treatment outcome.

When it comes to improving comfort during microneedling, people with severe needle phobia may find that topical numbing creams or even mild sedatives prescribed by a healthcare provider work well. Being open and honest with your skincare professional about your concerns and preferences allows for collaborative decision-making and tailored care delivery, which builds trust and promotes patient satisfaction.

CHAPTER NINE

ADVANCED METHODS OF MICRONEEDLING

COMBINATION THERAPY: PRP OR SERUMS COMBINED WITH MICRO NEEDLING

Combination therapy in microneedling involves boosting the results of the procedure with the use of specialized serums or Platelet-Rich Plasma (PRP), which is made from your blood and contains growth factors that stimulate the production of collagen and tissue repair. PRP is injected or applied topically into the skin after the procedure, amplifying the benefits of rejuvenation. Serums, on the other hand, can be customized to address specific skin concerns such as hyperpigmentation, acne scars, or aging.

These serums, enhanced with vitamins, antioxidants, or hyaluronic acid, go deeper into the microchannels made by microneedling, maximizing absorption and efficaciousness.

To perform microneedling with PRP or serums, the skin must first be cleansed and numbing cream applied if necessary. Next, a microneedling device with adjustable needle lengths is gently rolled over the skin, creating controlled micro-injuries. This process promotes the production of collagen and elastin, which in turn promotes skin regeneration. Following microneedling, PRP or serums are applied to enhance results. PRP is often injected into specific sites for targeted improvement, or spread throughout the treated area.

Carefully selected serums are then massaged or dabbed onto the skin, ensuring deep penetration into the microchannels. Post-procedure care usually consists of gentle cleansing and moisturizing, with specific instructions provided by your skincare professional for optimal results.

MICRONEEDLING TO RESTORE HAIR

This non-surgical method works for both men and women who are experiencing hair thinning or loss.

During the procedure, a specialized microneedling device with fine needles is rolled over the scalp, creating tiny punctures. These micro-injuries activate the body's natural wound-healing response, triggering the release of growth factors and stimulating dormant hair follicles. Additionally, this process improves the absorption of topical hair growth products, such as minoxidil or hair growth serums.

To undertake hair restoration with micro needling, the scalp must first be thoroughly cleaned; numbing cream may be applied to reduce discomfort; the micro needling device is then methodically moved across the scalp in horizontal, vertical, and diagonal directions; this ensures even coverage and stimulates the scalp uniformly; following the procedure, soothing serums or minoxidil may be applied to enhance follicle stimulation and promote hair growth; and, to maintain the health of the scalp, post-procedure care must include avoiding sun exposure and excessive perspiration.

Several weeks apart are usually advised for best results, with gradual improvements in hair thickness and density being noted over time.

BODY SCARS AND STRETCH MARKS: MICRONEEDLING

Stretch marks, which result from the skin's rapid stretching, and scars from surgeries or other traumas can both be visibly reduced with microneedling, a non-invasive procedure that creates microscopic punctures in the affected area that triggers the body's natural healing process and promotes the formation of new collagen and elastin fibers that smooth out the texture and color of the skin.

Stretch marks and body scars can be treated with microneedling which involves cleaning the skin, applying numbing cream if needed, and rolling or stamping the affected areas. This process creates thousands of tiny channels in the skin that can be penetrated by topical treatments like vitamin C serums or scar-reducing creams, which promote cellular turnover and collagen production, speeding up the healing process and improving skin elasticity. After the procedure, gentle skincare and sun protection are recommended, with the appearance of stretch marks and scars becoming more noticeable over time.

IMPROVING THE OUTCOMES OF MICRONEEDLING WITH PEELS OR LIGHT THERAPY

Depending on the type of skin and desired results, microneedling can be combined with chemical peels or light therapy to get even better results. Chemical peels, like glycolic acid or salicylic acid peels, exfoliate the skin's outer layer and improve the penetration of microneedling treatments. Light therapy, like LED or IPL (Intense Pulsed Light), further stimulates collagen production and reduces inflammation post-micro needling. These adjunct therapies can address issues like acne scars, uneven skin tone, and fine lines, enhancing the rejuvenating effects of microneedling.

To combine microneedling with peels or light therapy, the skin is prepared with a mild cleanser and assessed for suitability. A chemical peel may be applied either before or after microneedling, depending on the goals and condition of the skin. The peel solution is carefully selected based on its depth and the desired outcome, enhancing exfoliation and promoting skin renewal.

Alternatively, light therapy sessions are performed right after microneedling to calm the skin and boost collagen production. LED light therapy, for example, uses specific wavelengths to target different skin concerns, promoting healing and enhancing the results of microneedling. For best results, multiple sessions of light therapy are advised following microneedling.

ADVANCED TREATMENT PLANS AND CASE STUDIES

Microneedling case studies and advanced treatment plans provide real-world examples of patient outcomes and customized approaches for particular skin concerns. The versatility and efficacy of microneedling in treating conditions like acne scars, aging skin, and hyperpigmentation are demonstrated by these studies.

Advanced treatment plans include personalized protocols that may involve combination therapies, different needle lengths, and post-care regimens to maximize outcomes and guarantee patient satisfaction.

When examining case studies, skincare experts look at before-and-after pictures, treatment schedules, and patient testimonials to gauge how effective microneedling procedures are. These case studies show how customized treatment plans based on skin type, degree of concern, and desired results can be achieved with microneedling, and how advanced treatment plans can incorporate progressive sessions with deeper needles or the addition of adjunct therapies like PRP, serums, or peels to achieve complete skin rejuvenation.

By recording and disseminating successful case studies, practitioners inspire and educate their patients while demonstrating the revolutionary potential of microneedling in aesthetic dermatology.

CHAPTER TEN

TROUBLESHOOTING AND TYPICAL ERRORS

MANAGING INEFFECTIVE TREATMENTS OR UNSATISFACTORY OUTCOMES

If the results of microneedling are not up to par, the first thing to do is evaluate the depth and frequency of the needle penetration. Inexperienced practitioners frequently make the mistake of applying too little pressure or not covering the treatment area evenly. If these factors are checked and results are still not up to par, the type of serum or topical used after treatment should be taken into consideration as the incorrect product may not effectively enhance the microneedling effects.

Inadequate skin preparation is another common problem. It is important to clean the skin well and use an appropriate antiseptic to prevent infections. Retinoids and sun protection should also be part of pre-treatment routines.

Post-treatment care is also important; using gentle, non-irritating skincare products can help soothe the skin and promote better healing and results. If these steps are not followed, the results may be disappointing.

Last but not least, the state of the microneedling device is important. Make sure the needles are sharp and that the device is sanitized thoroughly before each use. Needles can be blunt over time, which decreases their effectiveness. Frequent maintenance and prompt needle replacements guarantee that the device operates at peak efficiency and consistently produces the intended results.

RECOGNIZING ADVERSE EFFECTS OR ALLERGIC REACTIONS

Detecting allergic reactions or side effects from microneedling requires close monitoring of the skin's reaction after treatment. Mild swelling and redness are typical, but more severe reactions, like prolonged redness, excessive swelling, or itching, could be an indication of an allergic reaction. Keep an eye out for any odd feelings or changes in the skin, and act quickly if these symptoms don't go away.

Patch testing, which is a proactive measure, especially for those with sensitive skin or known allergies, can help prevent allergic reactions. Apply a small amount of the product on a discrete area of the skin and wait 24 hours to observe any adverse effects. If no reaction occurs, it's generally safe to proceed.

This approach helps mitigate the effects of adverse reactions and ensures safe and effective microneedling practices. If an allergic reaction or adverse effect is suspected, discontinue all products and treat the area with a gentle.

ADAPTING THE METHOD TO INCREASE COMFORT AND EFFICIENCY

You can achieve optimal results with minimal discomfort by adjusting your microneedling technique. To begin, make sure the depth of the needle is appropriate for the treatment area.

Shallow depths work well for delicate areas like the eye area, while deeper penetration may be required for thicker skin areas like the forehead or cheeks.

To cover the entire area uniformly, move the device in a systematic manner (horizontally, vertically, or in a cross-hatch pattern). This will prevent overlapping and ensure that every part of the skin receives equal treatment, which will promote better overall results. Another important thing to remember is to maintain a steady hand and use consistent pressure.

Another important consideration is when to time your treatments. Give the skin enough time to heal and regenerate between sessions; too little time can cause irritation and reduce results; too much time can cause under- or over-reactions; a normal interval lasts four to six weeks, depending on the goals of the treatment and the response of the skin. By adhering to these guidelines, you can maximize comfort and effectiveness.

TYPICAL ERRORS MADE BY NOVICES AND SOLUTIONS TO PREVENT THEM

Sterilizing the microneedling device before use is a common mistake made by beginners. This can result in infections and other complications. To prevent contamination and maintain hygiene, sterilize the needles with isopropyl alcohol before and after each use.

Overzealous application can cause unnecessary skin trauma, leading to irritation and longer healing times. It's important to use a light, consistent hand and let the device do the work. Microneedling should be a controlled and gentle process to avoid damaging the skin. Using the device too aggressively or applying too much pressure is another common mistake.

Ignorance of proper post-treatment care is another common mistake made by beginners. Following microneedling, the skin is extremely sensitive and requires gentle care.

INVESTIGATING EQUIPMENT PROBLEMS

First things first when troubleshooting microneedling equipment malfunctions: make sure the device is charged or has new batteries. Insufficient power is a common problem with electronic microneedling devices, which can cause the device to stop working mid-treatment. Checking the power source regularly can help prevent unplanned interruptions.

Another crucial step is to check the needle cartridge to make sure there are no bent, broken, or dull needles, as these can reduce the effectiveness of the treatment and possibly cause damage to the skin. If there are any signs of wear or damage, replace the cartridge right away, as using a damaged cartridge can worsen the situation and put you at risk for injury.

Following the manufacturer's instructions for care and maintenance will extend the device's lifespan and guarantee that it operates correctly every time.

CHAPTER ELEVEN

NEXT DEVELOPMENTS IN MICRONEEDLING

TECHNOLOGICAL ADVANCEMENTS IN MICRONEEDLING

Modern aesthetic dermatology has experienced a revolution in microneedling technology, bringing about more effective and accessible procedures than ever before. Among the major innovations are automated microneedling devices, which provide exact control over needle depth and speed, guaranteeing consistent results for various skin types and treatment areas. These devices not only shorten treatment times but also minimize patient discomfort and downtime, making microneedling an attractive option for people with busy schedules who want to rejuvenate their skin.

The incorporation of radiofrequency (RF) energy into microneedling treatment devices represents advancement in the field.

RF microneedling is a combination of traditional microneedling and the advantages of RF therapy, where heat is delivered deep into the skin layers to stimulate collagen production and tighten the skin. This dual-action approach improves outcomes for patients with wrinkles, fine lines, and skin laxity, providing a non-invasive alternative to more invasive procedures.

Additionally, improvements in the design and composition of needles have increased the safety and effectiveness of microneedling treatments. Ultra-fine needles composed of premium metals, like titanium, minimize skin trauma while optimizing the absorption of topical serums or PRP (platelet-rich plasma) during treatments. These developments highlight the continued dedication of dermatologists and researchers to improving microneedling technologies and techniques, which will ultimately improve patient outcomes and satisfaction.

DEVELOPING APPLICATIONS FOR MICRONEEDLING

Beyond its initial use for rejuvenation of the face, microneedling is now being used to address a wide range of dermatological issues and aesthetic objectives. One new use for microneedling is the treatment of acne scars; in this case, the technique is especially helpful for people with acne-prone skin who want non-ablative treatments with little downtime because it breaks down scar tissue and stimulates collagen production to gradually improve skin texture and appearance.

Microneedling is a rapidly expanding field that offers a non-invasive alternative to surgical hair restoration procedures for both men and women experiencing mild to moderate hair loss or thinning hair. By creating microchannels in the scalp, microneedling encourages blood flow to hair follicles and promotes the absorption of hair growth serums, ultimately leading to thicker, healthier hair growth.

Additionally, as research into new applications and combinations continues, microneedling remains at the forefront of innovation in aesthetic dermatology, offering adaptable solutions for a wide range of skin concerns. Combining microneedling with other cosmetic treatments like PRP therapy or topical vitamin-infused serums enhances the overall efficacy of microneedling by delivering beneficial ingredients directly into the skin through the microchannels created during the procedure.

STUDIES AND ADVANCEMENTS IN SKIN REJUVENATION

Microneedling techniques for natural healing and rejuvenation have advanced due to ongoing research and development in skin regeneration. One area of focus is the use of growth factors and cytokines to enhance the regenerative effects of microneedling; these bioactive substances improve skin elasticity, stimulate collagen production, and speed up the healing process, ultimately resulting in smoother, more youthful-looking skin over time.

Research on biocompatible materials for microneedle fabrication is another promising area of study. Targeted treatments can be delivered to specific layers of skin with biodegradable microneedles loaded with stem cells or therapeutic agents, maximizing effectiveness and reducing side effects. These developments highlight the potential of microneedling as a therapeutic tool for dermatological conditions, including pigmentation disorders, scars, and even chronic wounds.

Furthermore, as research into the complexities of skin regeneration continues, microneedling is poised to remain a cornerstone of non-invasive dermatological interventions, providing safe and effective solutions for improving skin health and appearance. Developments in imaging technologies, such as confocal microscopy and high-resolution ultrasound, have made it possible for researchers to visualize the microscopic changes in the skin following microneedling treatments. This deeper understanding of skin response mechanisms allows for more precise treatment planning and customization, ensuring optimal outcomes for patients with a variety of skin types and conditions.

TRAINING OPPORTUNITIES AND EDUCATIONAL RESOURCES

Since microneedling is becoming more and more popular, dermatologists, aestheticians, and other skincare professionals have had access to extensive educational materials and training opportunities. Accredited workshops and seminars provide practical instruction in microneedling techniques, covering important subjects like patient assessment, treatment protocols, and post-procedure care. The emphasis of these educational programs is on safety guidelines and best practices to guarantee the best possible results and patient satisfaction.

For skincare professionals looking to learn more about microneedling, online courses and webinars have also grown to be very helpful. These digital platforms offer flexibility and accessibility, letting learners study at their own pace and interact with knowledgeable instructors through interactive Q&A sessions and case studies. Typical topics covered include treatment customization, device selection, and the incorporation of adjunctive therapies like PRP or serums for better outcomes.

Skincare professionals can confidently integrate microneedling into their practice by investing in ongoing education and training. Professional organizations and medical societies devoted to dermatology also regularly host conferences and symposia that feature lectures and demonstrations on the latest advancements in microneedling. These events foster collaboration among peers and facilitate knowledge exchange on emerging techniques, clinical studies, and patient management strategies.

WORLDWIDE PATTERNS IN COSMETIC DERMATOLOGY

The field of aesthetic dermatology is currently facing several dynamic global trends that will impact the uptake and development of microneedling as a preferred non-invasive cosmetic procedure. Among these trends is the growing desire among patients seeking aesthetic treatments for results that look natural and minimal downtime; microneedling meets these needs by inducing the skin's natural healing processes without the need for surgical intervention, making it a popular option for those seeking gradual improvements in skin tone, texture, and firmness.

Globalization of beauty standards and skincare innovations: propelled by social media and digital platforms that present global aesthetic trends, microneedling has become more popular as a versatile treatment option for addressing a wide range of skin concerns in various cultural and geographical contexts due to this interconnectedness. Consequently, skin care professionals are modifying their practices to cater to the changing needs and preferences of a global clientele, emphasizing customized treatment plans and culturally sensitive skincare solutions.

Additionally, advancements in technology and accessibility have democratized aesthetic dermatology, opening up microneedling to a wider range of patients. The widespread adoption of microneedling in clinical settings and home-use applications can be attributed to innovations in treatment devices and techniques, as well as increased affordability and availability of skincare products. This trend toward democratization highlights the significance of evidence-based practice and patient education in guaranteeing safe and effective outcomes for individuals seeking microneedling treatments globally.

As the field continues to evolve, skincare professionals play a pivotal role in leveraging these trends to deliver personalized microneedling treatments that improve skin health, confidence, and quality of life for patients worldwide.